Turkey Necks and Humped Backs:

How Our Mobile Devices are Aging Us and What We Can Do about it in Three Easy Steps

Maxine Free

Copyright © 2015 Maxine Free

ISBN 978-1-63490-015-7

All rights reserved. No part of this publication may be reproduced, stored in a retrieval system, or transmitted in any form or by any means, electronic, mechanical, recording or otherwise, without the prior written permission of the author.

Published by BookLocker.com, Inc., Bradenton, Florida, U.S.A.

Printed on acid-free paper.

BookLocker.com, Inc.
2015

First Edition

DISCLAIMER

This book details the author's personal experiences and observations of the potential problems of a turkey neck and a humped back due to the prolonged use of hand held mobile devices. The author is a registered nurse, but has not worked directly for a chiropractor or a plastic surgeon.

The author and publisher are providing this book and its contents on an "as is" basis and make no representations or warranties of any kind with respect to this book or its contents. The author and publisher disclaim all such representations and warranties, including for example warranties of merchantability and healthcare for a particular purpose. In addition, the author and publisher do not represent or warrant that the information accessible via this book is accurate, complete or current.

The statements made about products and services have not been evaluated by the U.S. Food and Drug Administration. They are not intended to diagnose, treat, cure, or prevent any condition or disease. Please consult with your own physician or healthcare specialist regarding the suggestions and recommendations made in this book.

Maxine Free

Except as specifically stated in this book, neither the author or publisher, nor any authors, contributors, or other representatives will be liable for damages arising out of or in connection with the use of this book. This is a comprehensive limitation of liability that applies to all damages of any kind, including (without limitation) compensatory; direct, indirect or consequential damages; loss of data, income or profit; loss of or damage to property and claims of third parties.

You understand that this book is not intended as a substitute for a consultation with a licensed healthcare practitioner, such as your physician. Before you begin any healthcare program, or change your lifestyle in any way, you will consult your physician or other licensed healthcare practitioner to ensure that you are in good health and that the examples contained in this book will not harm you.

This book provides content related to topics physical and/or mental health issues. As such, use of this book implies your acceptance of this disclaimer.

This book is dedicated to everybody that uses a mobile device, especially the youngest of users – our next generation. 10% of the proceeds from the sale of this book and e-book will go into "Head Up/Chin Up" the educational program created by the author to teach children, teachers and parents the importance of good posture and healthy mobile device habits.

Table of Contents

Forward xi

Introduction 1

Chapter One: Times Have Changed 9

    Television Bumped to Number Two 12

    Everybody is at Risk 14

    Work/Play + Natural Law = Ergonomics 17

    The Alexander Technique 18

    Exercise One 19

Chapter Two: Turkey Neck – Tech Neck 23

    Cause of the Turkey or Tech Neck 24

    Loss of Muscle Tone 26

    Muscles 101: If You Don't Use It - You Lose It 28

    Exercise Two 31

    What Is Muscle Atrophy? 32

Chapter Three: The Humped Back – Kids Beware ... 35

    Causes of the Humped Back 37

Forward Arm Dangler 41

Typical Treatment for Humped Backs 44

Exercise Three 45

Chapter Four: Live in the Neutral Zone 47

What is the Neutral Zone? 49

The True Test – The Toilet Test 53

The Neutral Head Zone 56

The Neutral Shoulder Zone 58

The Neutral Hip Zone 60

Exercise Four 63

The Neutral Zone and You 64

Sitting in the Zone 65

Standing in the Zone 68

Chapter Five: Stretch and Strengthen for Daily Use 69

The Importance of Stretching 70

The Chin Press 74

The Neck Turn 76

The Ear Press	78
The Neck Roll	80
The Importance of Strengthening	82
Isometric and Isotonic Exercises	84
Strengthening Exercises to do Daily	86
The Chin Up	86
The Forward/Back Push	89
The Side to Side Push	91
The Chin Tuck	93
Chapter Six: Children and Mobile Devices	**95**
Exercise Five	99
Conclusion	**105**
Acknowledgments	**111**

Forward

Hand held mobile devices have changed the way we live our lives. Not only do we talk, socialize, shop and work on our hand held mobile devices, our devices are now teaching us about ourselves. The FitBit and other fitness wristbands are the newest mobile devices for adults. These devices tell us our heart rates, blood pressure, sleep patterns and daily calorie intake. As these devices assist in our health, they with the rest of hand held mobile devices may also have a negative impact on our health.

Hand held mobile devices have the potential of aging our bodies, if we are not careful. What our mobile phones, tablets, laptops and fitness bands do is force us to constantly look down. This motion of reading your text or shopping for those pair of shoes can easily lead us into the poor posture of hanging our heads forward, chin pressed to our chest and shoulders scrunched up. With a little bit of body awareness, the danger of poor posture on our mobile devices can be easily avoided.

Maxine Free

This book was written with the intention of introducing body awareness and the potential dangers of hand held mobile devices. Just as we take our daily multivitamin as a preventive tool, so to can this book be used as a preventive tool. A tool that can be used anywhere, at any time and by anyone – old or young. As a registered nurse, I have always been concerned with posture and how people hold themselves. Body mechanics is an important part of patient care and I have always included it in my nursing plans. But the nursing plans that dealt with proper posture were always for my older patients. If there were swallowing issues, I would check to see if they were hanging their heads down and chins pressed to their chest. If this were the case, I would teach the patient proper head posture and the importance of maintaining this posture. If they had difficulty breathing, I would educate my patients and their families on the importance of opening up their chest, shoulders back, head up, assisting their lungs with expanding and letting oxygen in. Back pain, hip pain, knee pain – the common pains for geriatric patients, can also be attributed to poor posture. Of course I am in no position to diagnosis or even suggest that their pain was due to poor posture. But, it is within my scope of practice to educate patients and their families on healthy living and wellness. Proper posture and how one holds oneself up for the world to see, plays a vital role in the overall health of our body and wellbeing, not to mention helping out some of those aches and pains we may be experiencing.

I've also been concerned with young children and their posture. It was usually centered on their heavy, ill-fitted backpacks that they carry to and from school. I remember seeing little kids lugging their overloaded backpacks to and from school. The backpacks would be hanging half-way down their legs, with their head, neck and shoulders straining way forward to balance out the heavy load. It appears that backpack makers have realized this problem and now have little backpacks for little people and larger ones for the rest of us. They have also made it much easier to adjust the straps, for proper fitting and some of them even have a waist strap for added support.

Today there is an even greater threat to children and their posture, and one that is threatening the very,

very young – video games and hand held mobile devices. Of course, the devices are not the threat. The threat lies in the amount of time they spend on their mobile devices and the potential of slipping into a more comfortable, less than desirable body posture, which is my main concern. Children are not in threat of turkey neck or a tech neck, but the possibility of a humped back is of great concern. Children's bodies are developing well into their late teenage years. Proper posture, strengthening and stretching needs to be a part of the lives of children and their mobile devices.

This would be a good time to mention my disclaimer. I have never worked in the field of plastic surgery, nor for a chiropractor. I have worked for many years in the healthcare field and have always been keenly aware of the body posture of my patients. This book is a product of my combined observations of hand held mobile devices and my observations of body mechanics of the young and the old. This book was created to be used as a preventive tool, with the hopes of preventing future problems of a turkey neck, tech neck or a humped back due to poor posture. If you feel you have a postural problem, or you suffer from headaches, insomnia, nerve tingling in your arms or fingers or you have pain of the head, neck or shoulders, please see your healthcare provider before attempting the stretches or exercises in this book.

Maxine Free RN

Introduction

The world of hand held mobile devices is a young world and still growing. Along with growth though, come the inevitable growing pains. This book will address an important and potentially dangerous growing pain within the mobile device world – poor mobile device posture. The issue is not our mobile devices or even the amount of time that we spend on them. The issue is how we hold our bodies, whether we are sitting or standing, as we check our email or latest bid. When people say that we should not spend so much time on our mobile devices and live a more balanced life, I would have to respectfully disagree. Mobile devices have become such an important part of our work, play, socializing and relaxing that our "balanced life" must include our devices. What needs to change is our awareness of our body posture on our hand held mobile devices. More specially, we need to be awareness of how we are holding our head, neck and shoulders as we use our mobile devices.

In a November 2014 Neuro and Spine Surgery journal called Surgical Technology International XXV, Dr.

Kenneth K. Hansraj, chief of spine surgery in New York City wrote an article called "*Assessment of Stresses in the Cervical Spine Caused by Posture and Position of the Head".* In his article he addressed the "billions of people using cell phone devices on the planet, essentially in poor posture". He goes on to describe the purpose of his study was "to assess the forces incrementally seen by the cervical spine as the head is tilted forward, into worsening posture". Dr. Hansraj also believes that fellow cervical spine surgeons need this data to have a more complete understanding in relation to the reconstruction of the neck. Dr. Hansraj also stated that after a review of the *National Library of Medicine* publications, there was no other study available to assess the stresses of the neck when incrementally moving the head forward.

What is interesting with Dr. Hansraj's article is that he is asking his fellow spine surgeons to consider their patients "forces incrementally seen by the cervical spine as the head is tilted forward". In other words, yes you can repair, reconstruct a cervical spine, but if their patient has continual poor head posture – perhaps that angle needs to be considered into your surgery. This is the same dilemma I also observed. The constant poor head and neck posture of the general public as they used their hand held mobile devices. So I decided that I needed to write this book based on three major, but subtle events that happened in the scope of a twenty four hour period. It was a Sunday morning and I was sitting at my kitchen table, first cup of coffee in hand. I started browsing through the most important part of the Sunday paper – upcoming sales. I noticed that at all the big named stores, there were large sections devoted to children, and I mean the very young children and mobile devices. Leap Frog, now has an entire Learning Library, for all ages. There is the Leap Frog Pad and Leap Frog Reader Books, there are not only tablets and mobile phones geared toward children, there is the Inno Tab, full of games and lessons, Nabi Tablets, Amazon Fire Kid edition and of course, all of the video games on Wii, PlayStation, Xbox and Nintendo. As the coffee settled into my gray matter, so did a glimpse into our future generation – a generation of incredibly bright people, operating their world remotely and efficiently from their mobile devices.

The second subtle sign appeared the next morning. I headed up to our local college and standing at the bus stop were about eight college students, all of them staring down at their hand held mobile devices. I did my business and returning home, I noticed the same eight students, hunched forward and down. I really don't think they even moved. I remember saying to myself, "ten years and you guys are going to be having hunched backs just like my seventy year old patients - guaranteed". The last and not so subtle sign came when I got stuck behind the Monday morning school bus. Every other block was stop and go, as I watched the children leave their homes and jump onto the bus. I couldn't help but notice some of the poor posture on these little kids. Their heads were pointing way forward, backs hunched out as they lugged their heavy backpacks. These little kids looked just like some of those seventy year old patients with poor posture, the hunched back and their forward heads pushing forward.

These were the final signs that motivated me to finally write about a subject that I think is very important – how we hold ourselves up in the world. As well as, address the issue of poor posture and our mobile devices. Good posture not only affects our appearance, our overall body structure and the appearance of being confident; it also affects things such as our joints, blood flow and our skin. For children it even has a more important effect on them, because their bodies are still developing, proper, strong posture assists children in healthy growing, healthy joints and strong muscles. You're never too young to learn proper posture, especially if mom and dad are practicing good posture along with you.

Practice puts brains in your muscles – Sam Snead

Chapter One: Times Have Changed will look at the increase of hand held mobile devices in our daily lives. Now more than ever people are banking, working, socializing, relaxing with a movie, or just killing time on their mobile devices. If healthy mobile device habits are not developed during these long stretches of time, risk of turkey neck or tech neck and a humped back is possible. The science of Ergonomics and the self-awareness tool of the Alexander Technique will also be discussed. Chapter Two: Turkey Neck – Tech Neck looks at just what does happen to the body when turkey neck occurs. We will address the most common cause of turkey neck, which is poor posture, over time, allowing the frontal neck muscles to become flaccid and weak. Tech neck, the modern day term for the same problem, is the result of poor posture, compounded by the long hours spent on mobile devices. In Chapter Three: Humped Backs – Kids Beware we will look at the fact that young children may not be interested in turkey neck, but they need to be concerned with the possibility of a humped back. This chapter will explore the most common cause of the humped back, which again are poor posture and the unique risks to our younger, still developing and growing generation. Chapter Four: Live in the Neutral Zone examines the very important, first of three steps that will help prevent a turkey neck, or tech neck and a humped back. Proper posture and being aware of your body throughout the day is the key to operating your mobile devices in a healthy way. Chapter Five: Stretch and Strengthen for Daily Use will explore why it is important to stretch and strengthen our neck muscles and tendons. Why stretching and strengthening is an essential part of preventing turkey neck, tech neck and humped back. Finally Chapter Six: Hey Kids Head Up/Chin Up will look at our children and mobile devices. The importance of the Neutral Zone, stretching and strengthening for their growing and developing bodies and the importance teachers and parents play in setting good examples of using their hand held mobile devices in healthy and productive ways. Throughout the book I have inserted exercises. These exercises give us the opportunity to try and test the topic that was just discussed. The underlying goal of these exercises though is to practice self-awareness of our body posture. To really feel how poor posture feels and then to feel the difference once it is corrected. It is this awareness of our body that will bring about the changes necessary to prevent aging from our mobile devices.

Dr. Hansraj wrote in his article that "people spend an average of two to four hours a day with their heads tilted over reading and texting on their smart phones and devices. Cumulatively this is 700 to 1400 hours a year of excess stresses seen about the cervical spine. It is possible that a high school student may spread an extra 5,000 hours in poor posture." (Surgical Technology International XXV)

It is those "extra 5,000 hours" written by a chief of spinal surgery that I believe this book is extremely important at this time. Our hand held mobile devices are not going anywhere, so we therefore need to learn to operate them in a healthy way. The three simple steps we will learn within this book are important, but there is an even more important role - as we practice these healthy mobile device habits throughout our day, we need to reflect and teach our children these habits as well.

Chapter One: Times Have Changed

Getting information off the Internet is like taking a drink from a fire hydrant – Mitchele Kaper

Our world has become a mobile world. Our hand held mobile devices are an important and integral part of our daily lives. If we are not texting, emailing or talking on our mobile devices, we are socializing, shopping or playing games. Mobile devices have moved into every part of our lives, with no end in sight. Mobile devices have also become an important tool for teaching our children. Children at younger and younger ages are able to learn computing, analyzing and organizational skills, thanks to Leap Frog and their Leap Frog Pad. It is this generation that will be taking mobile devices into the future. And it is this generation, most importantly that needs to learn healthy mobile device techniques.

The problem is not our hand held mobile devices. The problem lies in the sheer amount of time that people actually spend on their mobile devices. Most people are simply unaware of just how much time they are actually utilizing their devices. It was found in a recent study by eMarketer that people spend an average of 5 hours 46 minutes a day either online or on their mobile devices. What is remarkable about this April 2014 study is that for the first time in US history, people are spending more time on their mobile devices than they are in front of their televisions.

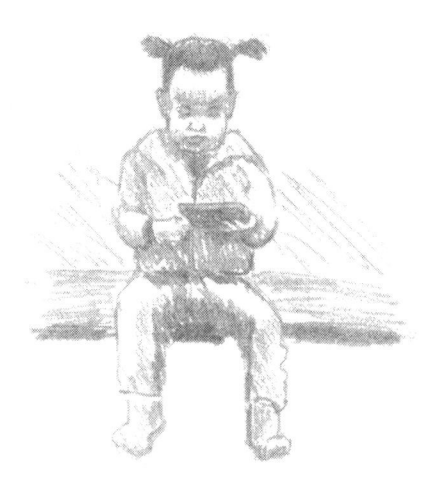

With these changing times of mobile devices, our knowledge and awareness must also grow with these changes. The changes are not only in personal growth through the technology that our mobile devices offer, but also within personal awareness and personal responsibility on our mobile devices. This book addresses the personal responsibility of good posture and a healthy balanced of mobile device usage. A good analogy would be when desktop personal computers first started entering households back in the 1980's. The keyboards were the standard straight, flat keyboards that we still see around, but nobody had discussed healthy PC techniques and proper body posture at that time. We realized pretty quickly that the old "hold your wrist straight and limb" for the typewriter could not transfer over to the standard PC keyboard body mechanics. Soon enough "carpal tunnel" reared its ugly head and thousands of people suffered permanent damage from improper hand posture on computer keyboards. Ergonomic keyboards are now available, so are wrist supports while working on your PC, padded key boards for wrist support, or good ole wrist braces that hold your wrists in proper posture. People now know that it was improper hand posture that caused carpal tunnel and that with wrist support, stretches and strengthening carpal tunnel can be avoided. I believe the same is true for poor posture and mobile devices and the long hours that we are spending on them.

Television Bumped to Number Two

As mentioned in the previous section the study from eMarketer found for the first time ever, digital media among US adults surpassed the time spent with televisions. To develop their figures, eMarketer analyzed more than five hundred data points collected from over forty research institutions. With respect to television, eMarketer looked and compared more than one hundred and forty data points from approximately thirty sources. What they found was that in 2013, US adults spent 43.4% of their time with digital media, as opposed to 37.5% watching television. In 2014 the gap grew larger with digital time clocking in at 47.1% and 36.5% watching television. Television has been bumped to number two! With the growth in apps and the convenience of down streaming movies and television programs, television watching just may stay in the number two spot.

The big difference between mobile devices and television watching is the fact that when we watch television, we are not staring down, watching the movie. With the conveniences of mobile devices, we can watch that movie anywhere, at any time but mobile devices force us to look down as we are watching that movie. Our television sets were placed at eye level and we kind of slouched into our couch, but we held our heads up because the television set is usually at eye level. Today we are so busy socializing, shopping or watching movies on our mobile devices; it is forcing some of us to stare down for hours at a time. The very convenience of our small, mobile devices force us to look down, chins pressed into the chest, hyperextending the back neck muscles and contracting the front neck muscles. What also happens is our shoulders slowly hunch forward and our heads hang down, slowly stretching out the natural curve of our cervical vertebrae. This comfortable, unconscious position is the perfect recipe for turkey necks, tech necks and humped backs. What took grandma and grandpa years to develop, we are developing in a fraction of time, all with the assistance of our tablets, phones and laptops, multiplied by the daily length of time we spend on them. Like the thousands of people that suffered from carpal tunnel after the introduction of the personal computers and keyboards. Hand held mobile devices could possibly injury many, if they are not aware of these potential problems and choose to develop healthy mobile device habits.

Everybody is at Risk

Chiropractors are seeing younger and younger patients suffering from kyphosis, also known as grandma's humped back. If there is one population that I hope really "gets" this book and understands and uses it as a preventive tool, it would be our children. Children develop and grow well into their late teen years. Dr. Hansraj the chief of spine surgery in New York City stated, "People spend an average of two to four hours a day with their heads tilted over reading and texting on their smart phones and devices. Cumulatively this is 700 to 1400 hours a year of excess stresses seen about the cervical spine. It is possible that a high school student may spend an extra 5,000 hours in poor posture". (Surgical Technology International XXV) I realize that this is the second time I have mentioned this fact from Dr. Hansraj's study, but I think it is so important, that it needs to be repeated! The high school age group is the group that practically lives on their mobile devices, whether it is homework, socializing, or playing video games, teenagers are at high risk of obtaining the mobile phone hump. Not only do they use mobile phones and tablets, they lug those huge backpacks to and from school every day! If they are not consciously practicing proper posture, stretching and strengthening their neck and back muscles, they are going to be looking like the hunched back of Notre Dame before their adult years.

Maxine Free

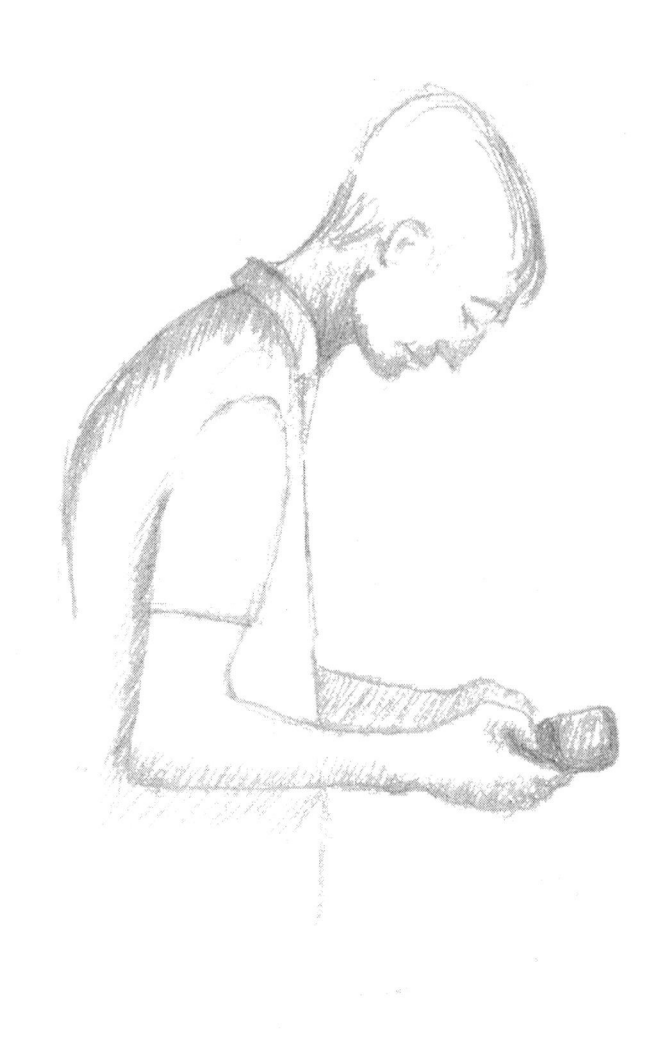

Work/Play + Natural Law = Ergonomics

The study of Ergonomics comes from two Greek words - "ergon" which means work and "nomoi" meaning natural law. Ergonomics is becoming more popular these days due to our new technical world and the strain it is causing our bodies. Ergonomic stores are popping up everywhere offering people devices, tips and equipment for maintaining that "natural law" of our body.

The field of Ergonomics is booming and developing more and more products for healthy body mechanics in the work place and for the home. But the ergonomic field has not been able to keep up with the exploding business of mobile devices. Businesses are also sprouting up everywhere, assisting people with chin lifts, mini facial lifts, surgically correcting the turkey neck syndrome. This is also a booming business and in my opinion, for a preventable problem. Being aware of your body during the times you spend on your tablets or mobile phones, is a powerful tool of prevention. Ergonomist have adopted a technique called The Alexander Technique which is "a simple and practical educational method which alerts people to the ways in which they are misusing their bodies, and how their everyday habits of work may be harming them." www.ergonomics.org.

The Alexander Technique

The Alexander Technique was devised by an Australian actor, Frederick Matthias Alexander. Alexander suffered from *globus hystericus,* or voice loss when on stage. Alexander was a keen self-observer and realized that when he even thought about performing on stage, he would lose his voice. Alexander observed himself in a three-way mirror and noticed that he automatically pulled back his head and tightened his throat muscle when he thought about going on stage. He saw how unconsciously his posture, balance and even the movement of his body changed with these thoughts. He consciously corrected his head and neck positions and felt his voice relax. Even though this new stance felt odd, he persisted and with it a new confidence and a strong, stage voice was born. Alexander spent nine years studying his body and the body posture of others. He observed that "the head, neck, and upper and lower back must be in dynamic equilibrium with each other for maximum lengthening of the spine and optimum energy and health". (www.ergononics.org) The Alexander Technique also offers other benefits such as:

- Always being aware of the position of your head, neck and spine
- Revealing bad postural habits
- Gaining freedom of movement with the correct use of your body
- Being aware of undue tension and stress in your muscles
- Preventing damage to your body due to bad habits and poor posture

Exercise One

As you are reading these very words, are you aware of your posture? Is your head hanging forward and down? Is your chin pressed against your chest? What about your shoulders? Are they slouched forward and up towards your ears? Is your gut kind of sticking out? This is the usual, relaxed, kind of unconscious and comfortable posture our body slips into when we are reading the newspaper, or spending hours on our hand held mobile devices. Now let's apply the Alexander Technique and have your "head, neck and upper and lower back in dynamic equilibrium for optimal energy and health". Hold your chin up, parallel with the ground; tuck it in toward the back of your neck and not sticking out forward, ears aligned with your shoulders. Lift your device or this book up to eye level, placing your shoulders down and back, tummy in. Can you feel the difference? Good posture is one of the three simple steps that we will learn about in this book.

Not only is the field of Ergonomics and cosmetic surgeries booming, skin tightening creams and other expensive cosmetic neck creams are finding their way onto the market. I recently saw an advertisement for

NIA 114 technology StriVectin cream, it claims to be the only #1 neck cream stating that "you're only as young as your neck" and that the NIA-114 Gravitite –CF Lifting Complex, TL Advanced Tightening Neck Cream "restores skin's elastin architecture for a beautifully contoured, youthful profile". This StriVectin cream claims to tighten skin, improve firmness and significantly lift the neck. I believe this book could also make these same claims using what people already have, the muscles in their own neck.

Since we are on the topic of facial skin, I would like to bring up some food for thought. Just think about the habit of always looking down at our hand held mobile devices. Not only does this constant looking down affect our necks and upper backs, but think about the bags under our eyes. With our heads constantly hanging down, does extra fluid and skin gather under our eyes, and around the mouth? What about the frowns on our forehead? Does the constant looking down assist those forehead lines with growing deeper and deeper? Let's stop aiding gravity with aging us. With these three, small steps – good posture throughout the day, stretching and strengthening our necks, we do not have to be the victims of turkey neck or the humped back. These simple three steps, which should take less than ten minutes a day, will also help reduce neck and back pain, headaches, stress and strain.

Chapter Two: Turkey Neck – Tech Neck

If it keeps up, man will atrophy all his limbs but the push button finger - Frank Lloyd Wright

The first time I ever heard of the term turkey neck was when I walked in on my mother getting ready for bed. I was probably thirteen or fourteen and she was untangling her new chin strap that had just arrived. She was really excited to try it on and I remember trying to wrap my brain around the idea of strapping in your chin before bed – it just didn't make sense. She explained that her Sears catalog had promised that this strap was going to help her with her turkey neck and all she had to do was strap in her chin every night. She explained that I would understand when I got older, but unfortunately the memory of her chin and head all strapped up, is just a confusing memory that has been seared into my brain. Since that impressionable age, I just accepted the fact that turkey necks happened to women when they got older and that's why they have to wear turtlenecks or scarfs.

Of course I know better now. She was participating in the latest fad to deal with a problem that appears to be a sign of old age. These days it seems that more and more businesses are popping up helping the aging adult with their turkey necks. Not only do they still claim that straps may help a turkey neck, there are now special creams and serums, there is an array of surgeries, Botox injections and skin lifting procedures. The market is growing for the treatment of turkey neck and it appears as the baby boomers become older, the more variations in treatment appear. With a new generation of tech necks coming into age, it'll be interesting to see what new treatments are developed for their turkey necks and computer humped backs.

Cause of the Turkey or Tech Neck

As a medical professional, I know that turkey neck is not a normal sign of aging. There are several reasons why a person may end up with turkey neck, for example genetics can play a part, or a certain body structure can cause turkey necks. For the purpose of this book though, we are going to focus on one of the most common reasons why turkey neck happens. It is basically the result of poor posture which continued over time. The law of gravity states that if you're looking down, eventually those body parts will follow. The neck unfortunately has to follow the head and will hang forward and down also. Why should we help gravity age us? The effects of gravity are the same for both men and women – the saggy skin and wrinkles under the chin. Sometimes it is clear to see there is no more muscle mass in the neck. This is when the neck appears "chordy". A chordy neck is the result of poor posture and poor muscle tone. The small frontal neck muscles become flabby or wasted away, therefore the tendons underneath are more visible and appear to be protruding from under the skin. Or if you are in the habit of holding your head way forward and out, this stretches and strengthens those tendons, forcing them to appear chordy under your neck skin.

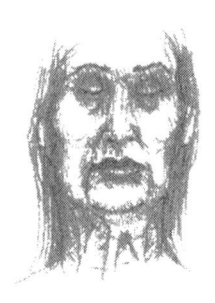

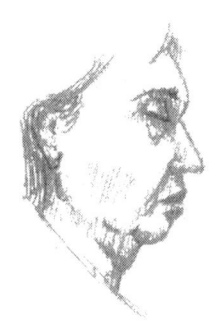

The neck is such a small area, with small muscle groups and the tendons are very strong and easily show through our thin skin. When we aid gravity, the frontal neck muscles are not used and muscle atrophy sets in due to this lack of use. Muscle atrophy decreases muscle mass in the neck and the lack of muscle mass causes lack of muscle shape and tone.

Loss of Muscle Tone

When we are aiding gravity and not using our neck muscles for their intended purpose, the largest frontal neck muscle – the platysma loses its tone and strength. When muscles lose their tone or shape, they also lose their ability to burn fat efficiently. And when muscles fail to burn fat cells, fat begins to deposit and to accumulate into fat pockets on and around the neck. Over time, with these fat cell pockets, the skin sags because of the flaccid muscle tone and lack of support. Wrinkles and sagging skin set in and a turkey neck is born.

The good news is turkey neck or tech neck, as a result of poor posture, is totally preventable. Being aware of what good posture, especially during times of reading, writing or using your hand held mobile devices, is one of the keys. The other two steps we will also learn about – stretching and strengthening – help keep the neck muscles long, strong and lean. These three steps will decrease the risk of neck muscle atrophy. Muscle atrophy as defined by *A Woman's Guide to Muscle and Strength* by Irene Lewis-McCormick, states that loss of muscle tone happens "as a decrease in muscle mass normally occurring as a result of disuse following prolonged immobilization. With muscle atrophy, fat levels increase but with increased resistance of muscles, this process can be reversed because muscle uses more calories and takes up less room than fat, diminishing fat stores."

Muscles 101: If You Don't Use It - You Lose It

Our neck is composed of many different small muscle groups with really big names like – the mylohyoideus or the geniohyoideus. Needless to say, these are typical skeletal muscles and if not used, say in the case of poor posture, they will atrophy, or deteriorate. The saying, "if you don't use it, you lose it" sums it all up. Here is some basic anatomy and physiology regarding muscles. According to my nursing book Medical-Surgical Nursing, 6th edition by Mosby there are three types of muscle tissue. There are the smooth (non-striated and involuntary) muscles that make up such things as our airway, our arteries and our gastrointestinal tract. We have no conscious control over these muscles, they work on their own. There are also skeletal (striated and voluntary) muscles that make up the majority of our muscles in our body. The skeletal muscles maintain our posture, assist in movement and make up all of the muscles groups in our necks. We have total control of these muscles and can make them move as we will. Lastly, there are the cardiac muscles (striated and involuntary) which are found only in the heart. These muscle tissues beat to their own drummer.

Muscles are composed of muscle cells which are highly specialized in order to produce muscle contraction. These muscle cells are made up of myofibrils, which consist of the contractile filaments called myosin, a thick filament and actin, which is like a thin filament. These are the basic building blocks of what makes a muscle cell contract and move. To produce a movement, a muscle cell contracts, causing the thick and thin filaments to slide past each other, causing the muscle cell to shorten and thereby causing a movement.

There are two types of contractions that make skeletal muscles move: isometric and isotonic contractions. Isometric contractions increase tension within a muscle, but does not produce a movement. Isotonic contractions shorten or contract a muscle to produce a movement. These two contractions keep muscles strong, toned and developed. In the chapter on stretching and strengthening, we will learn how to do both isometric exercises and isotonic exercise.

I once took care of a thirty year old woman who had been injured in a motorcycle accident. Her motorcycle had slid on some gravel and she went down, her bike fell on top of her right calf. She had pins holding her tibia and fibula, her calf bones, together as they healed. In the meantime, her right thigh muscles had atrophied, they had weakened and loss muscle mass. Her right thigh appeared to be one third smaller than her left thigh, because of this atrophy. With the help of a physical therapist, my patient learned how to do isometric exercises in bed. She couldn't bend or even move her right leg, so she had to learn how to apply resistance to her right thigh. This resistance – the isometric exercises – strengthened her immobile thigh muscles. She was providing resistance with her arms and pushing her right thigh against this resistance created by her arms. Every day she did her isometric exercises, and her right thigh became stronger and her muscle mass returned.

Exercise Two

Have you ever said to yourself during a workout, "after my crunches here, I'm going to work out my neck?" Nobody really thinks about their neck and their neck muscles unless they are a professional trainer or a body builder. The truth of the matter is that most of us tend to ignore our necks, until we don't like the sight of it anymore and then it seems that plastic surgery or turtlenecks are our only options. In this exercise we are going to utilize the Alexander Technique and become aware of the small area of your body known as the neck. Our skinny, little neck, with this heavy mainframe of a head sitting on top of it, how does it feel at this moment? Are the muscles tense? Sore? Does your neck stick out forward? What about when you are driving? Is your head sticking way forward, away from your body? What about your children?

When they are sitting at the table, or a desk, do they hold their heads forward, neck straining away from their body? Let's begin to become very aware of the posture our upper body, our shoulders, our head and how we hold our head. Bring your head back and up. Align your ears over your shoulders, alleviating the stress of the neck – do you feel the difference? Can you maintain this throughout your day?

What Is Muscle Atrophy?

Muscle atrophy is defined as "the wasting of muscle, characterized by decreased circumference and flabby appearance leading to decreased function and tone. The etiology or cause is the contractive, prolonged disuse as a result of immobilization." (Gray's Anatomy 6th edition)

The muscles in the neck react largely in the same way as the definition of muscle atrophy given in Gray's Anatomy. If we practice poor posture, with our heads hung down or forward, chins pressed into our chest, those frontal neck muscles are not being used properly nor strengthened. People associate turkey neck with aging because it is most often seen in older adults. It took years of poor posture to develop their turkey neck. With the introduction of hand held mobile devices and time spent on them, there is a potential of the same effect happening at a much faster rate. Mobile devices have the potential for aging the neck more quickly because people have a tendency of holding their devices much lower than one would hold a book or a newspaper for example. Some people stand or sit and hold their devices below their waist, forcing their heads to hang even lower. As the head hangs lower away from its center, which is squarely over the shoulders, the actual weight of the head increases. Have you ever tried to lift something heavy by just bending over and trying to lift it? Can you feel your back muscles scream in pain? Can you feel the ligaments in your back tear, causing even more damage? That's because when you bend at your waist – away from the center of our body – the weight of the body at that angle increases, adding to the weight of that heavy object. Now if you stay within the center of your body, keeping your back straight, bending at the knees and then picking up that heavy object – no problem, no damage done! The exact natural law applies to the neck. We will discuss this natural law of body mechanics and its implications later on.

Chapter Three: The Humped Back – Kids Beware

Some people say video games rot your brain, but I think they work different muscles that may be you don't normally use - Ezra Koenig

Our heads weigh roughly ten to fifteen pounds, the weight of a bowling ball, and sits on the smallest and most complex part of the spine, the cervical vertebrae. It is these cervical vertebrae that house all the nerves that come up from the entire body. A good analogy with the body, neck and head is to think of a complex super, multi-lane highway. This super highway, our bodies, house miles and miles of nerves, nerve endings, blood vessels, the lymph system, muscles, tendons and ligaments. All of these systems come up through the neck, narrowing down to one single lane as they pass by the cervical vertebrae, on their way to the brain, our mainframe. That one lane road is the area that is responsible for keeping that fifteen pound ball up and straight. When our mainframe head constantly hangs down, chin pressed to the chest, the single lane road has a serious bend in it and all of those bodily systems are also crimped and bent. It makes you wonder what information, impulses or important circulating nutrients are backing up in that crimped bend in the road? Are there any long term negative effects? Only time will tell.

Poor upper posture basically consists of not maintaining the natural balance of the spine and head. When we read or write, our heads move from the naturally balanced position of sitting squarely over the cervical vertebrae and our shoulders, to a comfortable, but unnatural position of hanging down and forward. Our chin is pressed into our chest, our shoulders hunched over and our upper back slouched. Our fifteen pound bowling ball, being held up by the small muscles and tendons that make up our neck, then places great stress and strain on the back of our neck and upper back muscles. Meanwhile, the frontal neck muscles are continually scrunched together, contracted and underused. When we are unaware of this poor posture, over time the frontal neck muscles are continually in a state of contraction and begin to atrophy. The posterior or back neck muscles are in a constant state of hyper-flexion and being overstretched. Another analogy would be to think of a golf ball sitting on top of its tee, the golf ball being the head and the tee reflecting our thin little neck. If our head, the ball is not sitting straight up on its tee, what happens? Of course, our head is not going to fall off because of our tendons, ligaments and muscles, but you get the point.

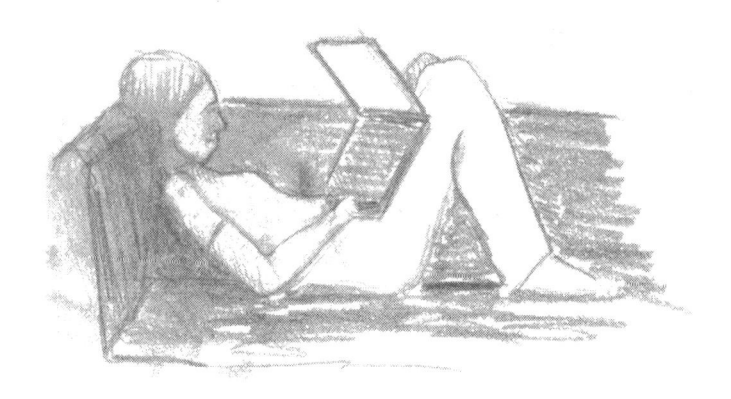

Causes of the Humped Back

As with turkey neck, a humped back is not a normal part of the aging process. Humped back is also known as kyphosis, which is the rounding of the thoracic vertebrae. According to the Mayo Clinic, the humped back can happen at any age, but is usually seen in older women due to a decrease in estrogen. This usually happens over time and usually because of poor posture. With poor posture, the vertebrae compress against each other, causing a wedging effect and a hump develops in the thoracic vertebrae, the upper back.

Humped back also occurs for other reasons, it could be congenital or a birth defect or caused by trauma or an injury or a humped back could be the result of a disease. The most common cause of a humped back though, is due to poor posture. This book will only focus on the postural causes of a humped back. In fact, kyphosis is now seen in younger and younger patients. This is due to the invention of video games, hand held mobile devices and the many hours spent on them. Children are especially prone to slouching over as they play for hours on their video games. A chiropractor in Florida by the name of Dean L. Fishman D.C., coined the phrase "text neck" based on all of the young patients that were showing up for treatment at his office. He defined text neck as "an overuse syndrome or a repetitive stress injury, where you have your head hung forward and down looking at your mobile device for extended periods of time." He goes on to say that "the human head weighs approximately 10 lbs. and that for every one inch of forward head posture away from neutral, the weight of your head increases by 100%." Dr. Fishman mentions on his website that he has recently had to treat a three year old patient. This little girl was constantly using her iTouch pad to play games. Her mother noticed that she was suffering from headaches and neck pain and brought her into Dr. Fishman's office for treatment.

So what happens when we are continuously hunched forward, head hanging down, glued to our Facebook page? Kind of the opposite of what happens to the front of the neck, except it includes the cervical and thoracic vertebrae, also known as your neck and upper back. Instead of muscles contracting and becoming flaccid and un-toned, the posterior or back muscles of your neck and upper back are hyperextended and continually stretched. The tendons and ligaments are constantly over stressed and strained as it holds the head up for hours on end. This uneven continual stress on the cervical and thoracic vertebrae causes inflammation and eventually, over time, or over the many hours on our mobile devices, the vertebrae become wedged and a hump is developed.

Of course our wonderful bodies give us lots of warning signs before the inevitable hump. All of that stress that you hold in your neck is a warning sign. The pain, the headaches, tense sore muscle in the neck and upper shoulders are warning signs. It is our choice on whether or not we are going to listen and correct these warning signs, or if we are going to ignore them and continue on as usual.

If we continue to allow the constant overextension of the tendons, eventually the thoracic vertebrae are pulled out of their natural curve, causing a postural change or a humped back. This process can lead to osteoporosis, which was once thought of as a degenerative joint disease because it was usually seen in older adults. We now know that it is not a degenerative disease that happens over time. There are several causes of osteoporosis, but again this book will only mention one of the main causes, which chiropractors refer to as "mechanical stress". Mechanical stress happens when repetitive physical activities that cause cartilage deterioration, also known as poor posture during long hours of hand held mobile device usage. Another stress that is closely linked to poor upper mechanical posture is what I like to call the Forward Arm Dangler.

Forward Arm Dangler

The Forward Arm Dangler is closely linked with a humped back because it is a very subtle and common misalignment of our upper body. Forward Arm Danglers go through their day with their arms facing forward, palm of their hands facing the back, dangling their arms in front of their body. This poor posture is subtle in the sense that it entails a small forward rotation of our shoulders and wrists causing the thoracic vertebrae to hunch forward. The forward rotation turns our arms into a forward hanging posture as well, and we get Forward Arm Dangling. The reason this is closely linked with a humped back is because it feeds into the poor, forward hunching posture that can lead to a humped back. The way to correct Forward Arm Dangler syndrome is to move your shoulders down, away from your ears and back, turning your wrists to the side along your thighs. We will learn in the upcoming chapter that this simple movement is into your Neutral Zone.

Turkey Necks and Humped Backs

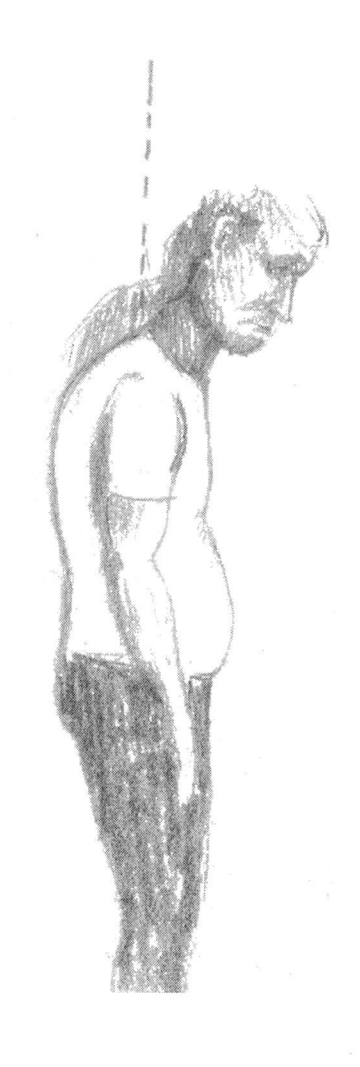

Typical Treatment for Humped Backs

Treatment for chronic kyphosis ranges from back braces, pain medication, anti-inflammatory medication, surgery or physical therapy. Dr. Fishman, the Florida chiropractor mentioned before, had a recent study on webpage. The study looked at two control groups that practiced a set of four specific exercises and both groups also receiving chiropractic adjustment. Except one of the groups was also asked to change their viewing angle of the phone as well, so they could comfortably see it, while holding it at a 90 to 70 degree angle from the floor. "Both groups improved, but the group that changed the angle did much better," explains Dr. Fishman "that was apparently the most important element". The key Dr. Fishman found, is strengthening and changing the way you're viewing your device. (See Dr. Fishman case study at text-neck.com)

In Dr. Hansraj's article *"Assessment of Stresses in the Cervical Spine Caused by Posture and Position of the Head"* the chief of spine surgery in New York's Spine Surgery and Rehabilitation Medicine states "cervical spine surgeons need to pay attention to the alignment and therefore to the stresses about the spine when performing anterior discectomies and fusion along with arthroplasties." He goes on to say how important the final position of the neck is stating "misalignment of a reconstructed segment into kyphosis will lead to a biomechanical disadvantage and more than likely will affect breakdown of the adjacent segment." What Dr. Hansraj is calling for is his fellow cervical spine surgeons to consider the patients forward head position and possible increased weight and stress on the spine due to poor posture and mobile device usage. He states in his discussion section of the article that, "as far as we are aware, and after a review of the *National Library of Medicine* publications, there is no other study available to assess the stresses about the neck when incrementally moving the head forward." (Surgical Technology International XXV)

Exercise Three

Using the Alexander Technique of self-awareness, how do you hold your shoulders? If you're able to look in the mirror, do your shoulders look like they are hunching forward? What about the placement of your arms? Do they hang forward, palms facing the back, in front of your body? Or are they placed to the side of your body? If you turn your arms so they hang along the side of your thighs, this small action rotates the shoulders naturally into a place of less stress – back and down. Turning your wrists to the side, palm of the hands facing your thighs also subtly rotates your shoulders into a place of less resistance. Can you feel the difference? Can you feel how heavy your arms feel when they are hanging in front of your body? Bringing your heavy shoulders forward as well? When they are placed along the side of your body, with your shoulders down? Can you feel the tension and stress leave? Do you feel stronger, having those strong, square shoulders in a neutral position with your head held high?

Chapter Four: Live in the Neutral Zone

Unless some misfortune has made it impossible, everyone can have good posture - Loretta Young

The Neutral Zone is the first, important step in the three steps of prevention of turkey neck, tech neck and humped backs. The other two that will follow are just as important, the stretching and the strengthening steps. The reason that the Neutral Zone is the first step is because it is the backbone, so to speak of prevention. It entails self-awareness. We will learn about the Alexander Technique, which is a self-awareness technique that can be done anywhere, and at any time. Self-awareness is the key to changing our body posture and instrumental in the prevention of problems, such as turkey neck and a humped back. If we are not aware of our body posture during our hand held mobile device usage, we will not be able to correct it. It is a very common mistake to simply lose track of time when we are busy with our hand held mobile devices. We simply are not aware of the total amount of time that we spend on them. After we check our email, texts or calls it's so easy to play a quick game of Candy Crush, check some posts on our Facebook, Pinterest, FourSquare, Twitter accounts, then check your latest bid on eBay. It is very easy for the time to slip away, unbeknownst to us. Whether we are standing or sitting, it is very easy for our bodies to fall into the comfort zone of poor posture. Because we are usually concentrated on our Candy Crush score, we easily ignore our body's warning signs of discomfort and pain.

Good, balanced posture helps people look and feel confident and outgoing. An article in TIME magazine by A.J. Cuddy called *Power Poser – Game Changers* discussed that "in proper alignment, spinal stress is diminished." Amy Cuddy and her associates went on to state that "[proper spinal alignment] is the most efficient position for the spine, and her studies have shown that high-power posture posers experienced elevations in testosterone, increases in serotonin, decreases in cortisol, and increased feelings of power and tolerance for risk taking". Interestingly, Cuddy and her team found that the "low-power posture poser", the people that exhibited poor posture with "the head in a tilted forward position and the shoulders dropping forward in a rounded position, exhibited the opposite pattern of the high-power posture people". Another point she goes on to mention about the low-power posture posers, is that it "leads to loss of the natural curve of the cervical spine, leading incrementally to stresses of the cervical spine, which may lead to early wear, tear, degeneration, and possibly surgeries." (Time.com)

What is the Neutral Zone?

The Neutral Zone is the zone of least resistance. It is the zone of the least amount of stress and tension being placed on your body, as well as the zone where your body is placing the least amount of stress on itself. The Neutral Zone is good posture at all times and begins with understanding the spinal column. The spinal or vertebral column is composed of 26 bone segments, called vertebrae, which are arranged in five divisions from the base of the skull to the tailbone. The first seven bones of the vertebral column form the neck bones and are called the cervical vertebrae (C1 – C7). These are very small and complex vertebrae that balance our twelve pound head. The second set of vertebrae is the thoracic vertebrae (T1 – T12). These twelve vertebrae make up our upper back and it is where the humped back is formed. The third set of vertebral bones is the lumbar vertebrae (L1 – L5). These five vertebrae are the largest and strongest of the vertebral column and make up the lower back. The sacrum consists of five segments of sacral bones that are fused together in childhood. The last division of the spinal column is the tailbone, or the coccyx and it is also fused and consists of four small bones. Between these vertebrae are intervertebral disks that act as a cushion against most shocks to the vertebral column and also aid in flexibility.

These five divisions of the spinal column are perfectly balanced. The cervical vertebrae curve naturally forward, balancing the weight of the head over our shoulders. Next are the thoracic vertebrae that balance the cervical curve, by curving naturally posterior or toward the back. The lumbar vertebrae curve naturally inward in the opposite direction, giving us that lower back curve and the sacrum and tailbones have a natural curve outward, giving us a tilt toward our hip bones and a natural sitting cushion. This is the

Neutral Zone. This is the zone that Mother Nature has created for our bodies to work and to play in. But what often happens is we become unaware of our body posture and we hang our heads forward, causing the cervical vertebrae to leave Mother Nature's natural zone, causing stress on the thoracic vertebrae as it fights to keep the head balanced. Or if we walk or sit with our lower spine curved too far out, it causes stress on our lumbar vertebrae, hips and knees. Our gut then tilts forward, to balance this posterior lumbar curve. These are examples of allowing our perfectly balanced vertebral column to operate outside of Mother Nature's natural zone, or the Neutral Zone.

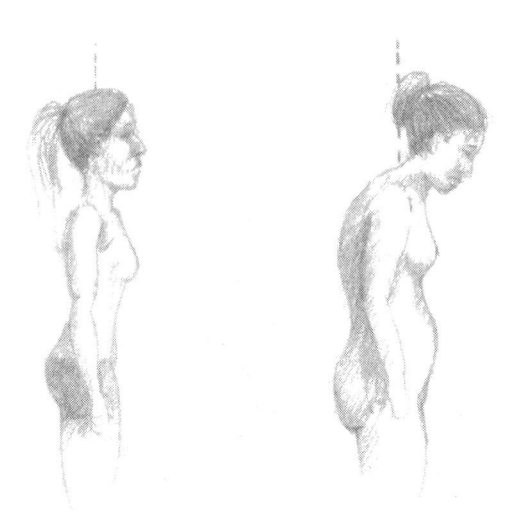

In the short term, these stresses are exhibited as neck aches, tight neck muscles, headaches, or lower back pain, hip or knee pain. If not corrected, or if we chose not to listen to these aches and pains, the long term effects are the chronic bone and joint issues such as arthritis, possible ligament or tendon tears, or fractures. With hand held mobile devices, the challenge of staying in the Neutral Zone and practicing good posture is even more important. The amount of time people are spending in the unnatural position of looking down and forward is increasing every year as mobile devices become smaller, more convenient and provide more services that are needed in our daily lives.

The True Test – The Toilet Test

I challenge you to take the true test – the toilet test. I call this the "true test" because this is where we are the most comfortable, and our most uninhibited selves, hence showing us our most comfortable body posture - on the toilet. The toilet allows us to be free from prying eyes and free from any social pressures. Whether you are the President of the United States, or just a kid, you can take the time to do the toilet test. The reason this is a perfect posture test is because we are so comfortable on the toilet and because we do our business and leave, so the time frame is short. Next time you visit your toilet become aware of your posture. Are you totally slouched over, head hanging down, shoulders hunched over? How is your spine? Is it totally curved outward, looking like a question mark? Or do you sit upright? Head held up? What about the waist? Do you lean way forward, bending at the waist, elbows resting on your knees? This small, brief moment can teach us a lot about whether or not we are prone to falling into poor posture, or whether we are aware of our posture, even in the most private and intimate times of our day. If you're prone to hunching over on the toilet, or bending at the waist and leaning forward on the toilet, you are probably prone to hunching over or leaning forward as you use your mobile device. With this awareness, correct your toilet posture. Sit straight up, shoulders aligned with your hips. Keep your head straight and looking forward as you do your business. If you must read that latest article while on the throne, hold it up to eye level. These small, incremental tests throughout your day will assist you and your proper posture throughout your other non-private moments.

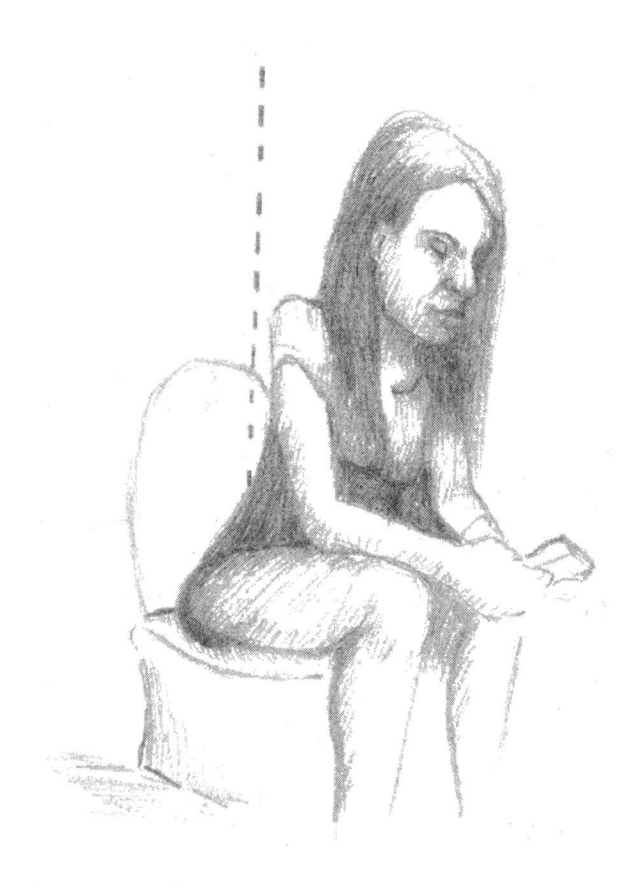

I have a confession - I do the toilet test all the time. Every time I do, I have to correct my poor toilet posture. Personally, I will sit on the toilet and hunch right over, shoulders forward, which by the way, is my go to lazy, comfortable poor posture I take when I'm reading, writing or just sitting. But I'm not done when I correct my poor toilet posture. This toilet time is the place where I do my neck stretches and strengthening that we will be learning about in the next few chapters. My toilet time is an excellent, private daily time to check into my posture and do my neck stretches and strengthening. Try it – it may work for you too!

The Neutral Head Zone

The Neutral Head Zone is the most important part of the Neutral Zone. Of course the entire Neutral Zone is important, but most people are not aware of the position that they hold their head in. We cannot really observe our own head, so therefore we are really not physically aware of the position of our head. This awareness comes from a conscious effort of awareness, or of applying the Alexander Technique. When we hold our head and neck outside of our Neutral Zone for long periods of time, our muscles and tendons start warning us. We start to feel tense in our neck or shoulders; maybe we have headaches or feel tension or pain in the back of our head. Often though, we are too busy or too consumed with the activities that we are doing to recognize these warning signs, let alone change them.

Our head is the first thing most people see. Okay, maybe it's our face, but our face is a part of our head, so it is really all one unit. Where our head goes, the rest of us will follow. Through sayings such as "head up, it's going to be fine", or she's "ahead" of her game, or "hold your head up high" we see how important our frontal unit or our head zone is.

There are mainly two improper, unhealthy head zone postures that people assume. One is the Forward Head Posture. The Forward Head Posture is common because we are a forward looking, forward moving species. All that we do is in the forward motion. The second common improper head zone posture is the Hanging Head Posture. Have you ever felt your head so heavy, especially if you've been sitting for a while, that you just have to rest your head in your hands? The head just hangs down, chin pressed into the chest especially when you are reading or texting? The Neutral Zone is the zone of least resistance and less work for the body. Your neck and head does not become exhausted in the Neutral Zone. As seen in Dr. Hansraj Surgical Technology International XXV article, *Assessment of Stresses in the Cervical Spine Caused by Posture and Position of the Head* the head weighs approximately 60 newton or 6 kg or 13.2 pounds. In the Neutral Zone, there is no stress placed on the neck or shoulders and the head maintains its average weight. But as soon as the head tilts 15 degrees, Dr. Hansraj states "the forces seen by the neck surges to 27 pounds". He goes on to state that when the head is at a 60 degree angle – chin pressed to chest, head hanging down – the weight of the head increases to 60 pounds! "These forces seen on the neck", the chief of spine surgery goes on to say "may lead to early wear, tear, degeneration and possible surgery".

The Neutral Shoulder Zone

The shoulders are our upper "check point". A check point is just that – a place where we can check in and know how our posture is at that moment. What makes the shoulders our upper check point and our hips the lower check point is because of the fact that they are centrally located. North and south, crosses with east and west making them our upper and lower check points. The Neutral Shoulder Zone consists of shoulders set back and, down. Most of us have a tendency of lifting our shoulders up, toward our ears. This lifting up adds stress and tension to our neck and shoulders. Open up that space between the ears and shoulders. Shoulders also have a tendency of falling forward, like our heads. The Neutral Shoulder Zone has the shoulders aligned with our lower check point – our hips. We have to consciously hold our shoulders back and down. When we are standing or walking are your arms hanging forward? This is a quick check that we can do.

More than likely, your arms are in front of your body, hanging forward, meaning your shoulders are hunching forward. Remember the Forward Arm Dangler syndrome? We have to remember to bring the arms back and align your arms with your thighs. This action of having your arms aligned with your thighs brings your shoulders back automatically. When you are in the sitting position, align your elbows with the lower check point, your hips and the same thing happens, your shoulders automatically go back and into the Neutral Zone.

The Neutral Shoulder Zone is a powerful zone because the act of bringing the shoulders back and down, automatically opens up the chest. With the opening up of the chest, we are able to inhale more oxygen, more of life in a productive way. But again this takes a conscious awareness of your body posture, with practice though, these healthy mobile device challenges become healthy mobile device habits.

The Neutral Hip Zone

The Hip Neutral Zone is important when you are standing, sitting or working on your hand held mobile devices. This lower check point is just as important as the upper check point, but dealing with the lower parts of our body and abdomen. The natural tendency of the body is to slouch over our mobile devices, causing our thoracic vertebrae to curve out and our lower vertebrae, our lumbar vertebrae – also known as our gut, to stick out, in the other direction, in order to balance the vertebral column. As our gut sticks out forward, we have a tendency to stick our butts out in the opposite direction, in order to balance the body. It's a chain reaction of poor posture.

The Neutral Hip Zone is picturing a line running along the side of our body, from the top of our head down to our feet. We have our ears over our shoulders and our gut tucked in, close to the line and our butt tucked in. People also have a tendency to lock their knees, pushing them back, especially if they are standing in one position for long periods of time. The knees should be slightly bent, along that invisible line.

In the sitting position, imagine the line from the top of your head, straight down through your chair. Your head is straight, chin tuck in and ears above shoulders. Shoulders down and slightly back. The tummy is tucked in toward the imaginary line, with your hips straight and not tilted outward. This position is going to feel awkward at first, especially if you have been unconsciously living in poor posture for some time. The ultimate goal is to stay in the Neutral Zone for as long as possible and as close to the Neutral Zone, for as long as possible. As with poor posture, good posture will happen over time and will become a healthy daily habit that you chose.

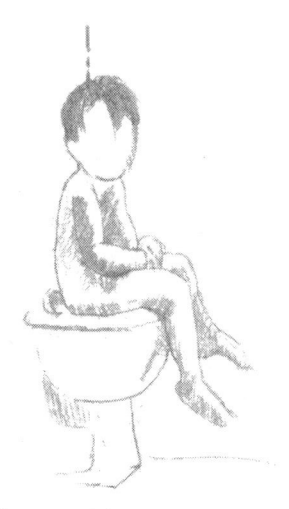

Symptoms of poor hip posture are the "over-the-belt-itis" also known as the "beer belly" or the "telly-belly", achy hips and sore knees. Living in the Neutral Hip Zone, will help tone the abdomen because you are aware of your stomach and tucking the stomach in. This will help strengthen and tone your abdominal muscles. With your body in its zone of least resistance, there is less wear and tear on the joints, especially the hips and knees.

Exercise Four

With the awareness of the Alexander Technique, does your body's posture follow an invisible line from head to toe? Are your head, shoulders and hips in the Neutral Zone? Beginning at the top of your head, image a line pulling your head up, chin tucked in. Do you feel taller? Do you feel stronger? Are your ears aligned with your shoulders? Or is your head leaning forward? With your head in the Neutral Zone, are your shoulders aligned with your hips? Or are they hunching forward? Following that invisible line down, are your arms hanging forward, or are they aligned with your thighs – in the Neutral Zone? Lastly, are your hips aligned with your ankles, or is your butt sticking out, with your stomach sticking out in the opposite direction? Tucking your butt in, with your stomach tucked in can you feel the difference of being in the Neutral Zone? What about your children? How do they carry themselves? Do they stand in the Neutral Zone?

The Neutral Zone and You

How does the Neutral Zone look like when you are using your hand held mobile device? The following section will review how the body looks like when it is using a mobile device in the Neutral Zone. Remember that this is the zone where the body is not producing any stress or tension on itself. It may feel different or awkward, especially in the beginning, but the body is happiest with the least amount of unnatural positions and stress is present. After some practice, the Neutral Zone and healthy mobile device habits will become second nature, and unnatural positions will feel painful, stressful and uncomfortable.

Sitting in the Zone

The science of mobile devices has exploded in recent years and the science of Ergonomics is lagging behind. So until the industry of accessories and proper mobile device support catches up, we are going to have to use items around the house to assist us. The goal of the Neutral Zone is for your spinal column to stay aligned. So make sure your back is properly supported, with a good chair or pillows. In order to avoid the Forward Head Position, or the hunching over of shoulders, we need our mobile devices at eye level and approximately eighteen to twenty-four inches away from our heads. Pillows or small blankets work well. Placing them on your table, desk or on your lap and kind of building them up to eye level. A stack of books also works well, but you will need the case for your tablet to be folded, so it holds your tablet up for you. With the pillows, you can make a kind of cubby hole for your mobile device to sit in and be supported.

Sitting on a sofa is the same idea, pile pillows or blankets up to eye level and tuck your mobile device in there. Or you can support your arms with pillows and hold your hand held mobile devices up in front of you and at eye level. It is important to remember to keep your shoulders down and back slightly – always checking your check points of shoulders over your hips and ears over your shoulders. Tucking your chin in will always get your head back, with your ears over the shoulders.

Turkey Necks and Humped Backs

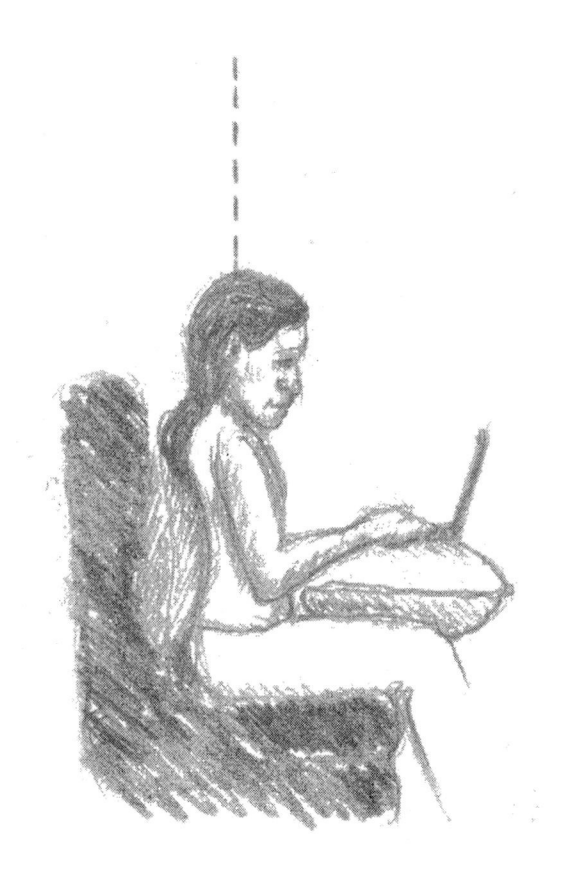

Standing in the Zone

For small children, it is difficult having them stand up straight and work on their mobile devices, holding it up to eye level. Supporting the devices on a book shelf, or on a counter, making sure it is supported and at eye level may work. Using a toy or stuffed animals may also work, if you can prop their mobile device up to eye level and supported by the toy. For older children and adults, remembering to keep the chin tucked in and ears aligned with the shoulders is the biggest challenge. The next challenge is using the arm muscles, bending at the elbows and lifting the mobile device up to eye level. It is not that difficult and keeping your elbows close to your body does add some extra strength. But it does feel different than just staring down at your hand held mobile device. Again keep in mind that your hips are in the Neutral Zone and your shoulders as well. When working out, or running remember to bring your wrist up to your eyes and read your FitBit wristbands. You may think, 'what's a couple of minutes looking down to read my heart rate?' But those couple of minutes really does add up in your total workout time.

Chapter Five: Stretch and Strengthen for Daily Use

Men have become the tools of their tools
- H.D. Thoreau

Staying in the Neutral Zone, especially when you are spending hours on your mobile devices is a very important key to reducing your risks of turkey neck and a humped back. Stretching and strengthening the neck muscles are also very important. As you learned in Chapter One, you want to keep your frontal neck muscles stretched, firm and strong. Not weak and neglected. These very short and very simple stretches and strengthening exercises will strengthen your neck muscles and will not bulk up your neck. To bulk up a muscle group, you have to put in long, repetitive movements with resistant weights. We will be doing no such thing here. The goal of this chapter is to introduce you to the importance of stretching our necks and gently strengthening the neck muscles. It is important to maintain muscle mass in our necks. You do not want your neck muscles to disappear, with your tendons protruding just under your neck skin. Also remember that muscles help burn up fat, so we need to keep our neck muscles developed, strong and lean.

The Importance of Stretching

There is a reason why yoga has become so popular. Of course it has many benefits, but one of its main secrets is the stretching. It is a well-known secret amongst the yogi masters that stretching one's body is the key to maintaining a young, healthy and vibrant body! Stretching helps circulate the blood supply to the muscle, helping in strengthen and healing that muscle and surrounding tissue. It also increases the rate and efficiency with which waste material is excreted from the body.

Stretching increases flexibility and prevents stiffness, tension and potential injuries. This is one of the keys of staying young - keeping your body moving, stretched and toned. Stretching also helps with range of motion in all of our joints and muscles. One of the most neglected parts of our body is our neck. People generally do not think of stretching or strengthening their necks. When working out the neck is considered, it is usually by body builders whose main goal is to bulk up that trapezius muscle group.

Stretching one's neck especially after long hours on your hand held mobile device can be heavenly. Those scrunched up, contracted frontal neck muscles will be almost singing to you, as you gently stretch them back and into the Neutral Zone! Some other benefits (besides singing muscles) are an increased range of motion in the neck, neck muscles and vertebrae of the neck. With this increase in range of motion and flexibility, comes a decrease in the risk of injuries to the neck. Improved posture will occur more naturally as there is less tension and stress in the neck. With well stretched muscles, comes the added advantage of preventing wrinkling and sagging skin, along with increased circulation of the muscles. With these added advantages, a boost in self-esteem and confidence naturally follows because nothing beats a well-shaped, chiseled looking jaw and neck line.

This list can go on and on. The benefits are almost endless but unfortunately, the lack of stretching can be debilitating and almost endless as well. As we learned in the last chapter, not stretching out your neck can cause muscle tension, tightness and weakness. If left over time, or over the many hours you spend on your mobile devices, it can progress to pain and permanent damage.

The following stretches can be done anywhere and at any time. I suggest that you do these stretches once a day. It would be kind of like taking your daily multivitamin, for preventive medicine. Personally I do these stretches and the strengthening exercises at the same time, in one sitting. And here comes my next confession…I do my neck stretches and strengthening exercises on the toilet. Yes, on the toilet. I do my toilet test, being aware of my sitting position and then I quickly do my neck stretches and strengthening and I'm on my way – done for the day!

Breathing during and between these stretches is also very important. We tend to hold our breath as we exercise or stretch. Breathing helps release tension and strain and helps the neck muscles to relax. Note: If you have or had any recent neck injuries or surgeries, please consult your professional healthcare provider before you begin these stretches and strengthening exercises. There are some points to remember when stretching - try not to bounce as you are stretching. Also if there is pain, listen to your body and stop the stretch. Always remembering to breathe during the stretches, stretch slowly and balance each stretch with the left and then right. Remember to keep your shoulders down, and not scrunched up to the ears and keep your shoulder blades slightly pulled back during each stretch.

Stretching Exercises to do Daily

The Chin Press

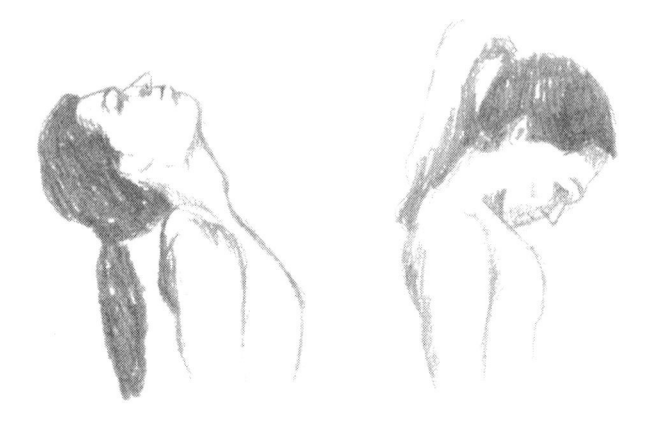

- **What is The Chin Press?** The Chin Press is an excellent stretch for your front and back neck muscles and tendons. As you breathe with this stretch, you will feel tension and stress leave the back of your neck and upper shoulders.

- **How do you do The Chin Press?** Sit up straight and in your Neutral Zone, slowly bring you chin down to your chest, breathe and hold this position for a count of ten. Bring your head back up, chin up looking at the ceiling, and breathe while you count to ten again. This is one set. Repeat this set three times.

- **Why is The Chin Press Important?** This stretch keeps the frontal muscles and tendons flexible and stimulated with blood circulation and movement. The strong back muscles are released of stress and tension.

The Neck Turn

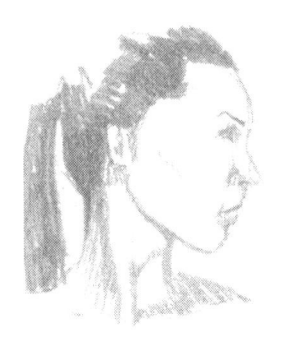

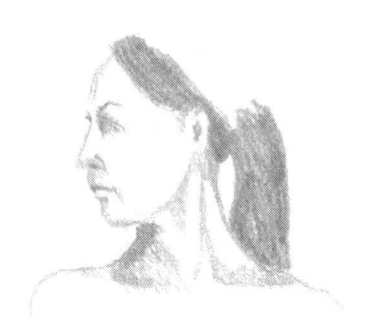

- **What is The Neck Turn?** The Neck Turn stretches the side muscles and tendons of the neck. This stretch aids in the lengthening the neck side muscles and preventing jowls development, which is a fat build up around our lower jaw.

- **How do you do The Neck Turn?** Sit up straight, spinal column strong and in the Neutral Zone, shoulders down and held squarely ahead, twist only the chin to the right, breathe and count to ten. Eyes should be looking right over the shoulder, chin up and parallel to the floor. Return to the center, breathe and turn your head over to your left shoulder, breathing and counting to ten. This is one set, repeat set three times.

- **Why is The Neck Turn Important?** Keeping our side neck muscles long and lean adds to a lengthened, well defined looking neck line.

The Ear Press

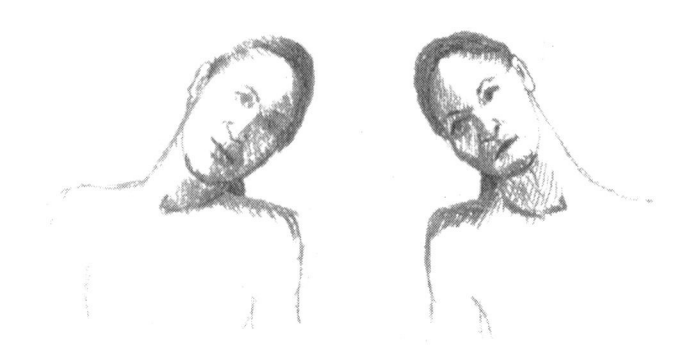

- **What is The Ear Press?** This wonderful stretch releases stress and tension held in our side neck muscles. The muscles that attach our neck to our shoulders also get a nice stretch.

- **How do you do The Ear Press?** In your Neutral Zone, shoulders down, press your right ear down as far as you comfortably can, toward your right shoulder, making sure that you don't lift your shoulder up.

Breathe and count to ten. Repeat on the left side, breathing and counting to ten. Be careful not to lean forward as you are pressing your ear down. This is one set, repeat the set three times.

- **Why is The Ear Press Important?** When we open up the space between our ears and our neck we create the ear canals to open up and drain more efficiently. This efficient flow happens to our jugular and other blood vessels, as well as our lymph and nervous system.

The Neck Roll

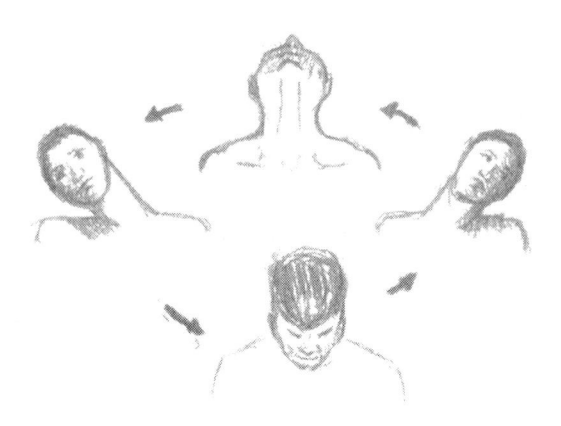

- **What is The Neck Roll?** The Neck Roll brings all of these stretches together. It allows for the superficial, large neck muscles to rub and roll over the deeper, smaller neck muscles and tendons, stimulating and causing them to move as well.

- **How do you do The Neck Roll?** This last stretch is bringing all of the stretches together. Starting in your Neutral Zone and remembering to breathe, with your shoulders down and not hunched up, bring your chin down to your chest and slowly roll your head to the right, then to the back, slowly to your left and then back to your chest. Slowly roll your head three times to the right, not forgetting to breathe and then repeat, rolling your head three times to the left. Try to feel all your neck muscles stretch, as you slowly roll your neck.

- **Why is The Neck Roll Important?** This is an overall stretch of the neck, neck muscles, tendons and associated chest, back and shoulder muscle stretch. It keeps them all vibrant and fed with fluids and blood that are needed for optimal muscle health.

- **Total Stretching Time:** 4 minutes

The Importance of Strengthening

In *A Woman's Guide to Muscle and Strength* by Irene Lewis-McCormick she states that strength training doesn't have to mean body building. She also discussed that resistance training is needed to increase their lean musculature, and decrease fat levels, stating that "the increased muscle diminishes fat stores by strengthening muscles, losing inches and creating strength".

These four, simple strengthening exercises will not bulk up your neck. To add muscle mass or "bulk up", you need to do massive amounts of repetition, with weights. We will simply be using our fingers to provide the resistant needed. So why is strengthening our muscles important? Strong muscles are on the frontline of protecting our bones, along with a healthy body weight, a healthy diet and a healthy lifestyle. Strong muscles help us maintain good posture, aiding us to be and look strong, confident and outgoing. Strong muscles, and again I do not mean bulked up and bulging muscles, but lean and toned muscles, are the best defense against aging. It burns up extra fat and keeps our skin firm and taut – which means less wrinkles and less sagging skin.

Especially in these days of mobile devices, we really want to keep in our Neutral Zone, with our neck muscles stretched and strong. As with the stretching, these four simple strengthening exercises can be done anywhere and at any time. I suggest that you do both the stretching and strengthening in one sitting. Don't forget to stay in the Neutral Zone. If you feel tension, tightness or any sort of pain in the back of your neck, you need to listen to your body! Are you working, playing on your hand held mobile device in the Neutral Zone? Next is to stop and take a few minutes to stretch and strengthen. Your neck and upper back will thank you and the turkey neck and humped back will stay away.

After you have stretched, your neck should feel a little more limber and flexible. Remember it is important to breathe through these exercises; we want to release any tension and stress your neck may be holding on to. Breathing is one technique that helps to release stress and muscle tension. With these strengthening exercises, we are going to add a very small amount of resistance with our hands. This resistance will help us build more lean muscle mass and help decrease the fat that may be storing up in your neck area.

Isometric and Isotonic Exercises

If you remember from Muscles 101, isometric contractions of the muscle increase tension of the muscle, but do not produce movement. Isotonic contractions shorten the muscle to produce movement. So it is the isometric exercises that produce tension in the muscle without the muscle being shortened or lengthened by actual movement. Therefore, the four strengthening exercises will consists of a combination of isometric and isotonic movements. Isometric exercises or Isometrics are a type of strengthen training in which the muscle length does not change during contractions. Isometrics are done in static positions, rather than actually moving. An isometric exercise is a form of exercise involving the static contraction of a muscle with resistance. This resistance can be a structured item, like a wall or a fence, or it can be one's own body, like our hands. The advantage of isometric exercise is that it can help geriatrics or bed ridden patients, build and maintain muscle strength and tone and prevent muscle atrophy. It can also strengthen and tone difficult to exercise places such as the neck.

Note: If you feel any pain or discomfort during these strengthening exercises, that is your body telling you that it is too much. Whether it is the angle, or number of repetitions, you need to adjust. Find the point where the pain or discomfort starts and stop there for now. In time, your neck will become more flexible and you will be able to do these exercises without any pain or discomfort.

Strengthening Exercises to do Daily

The Chin Up

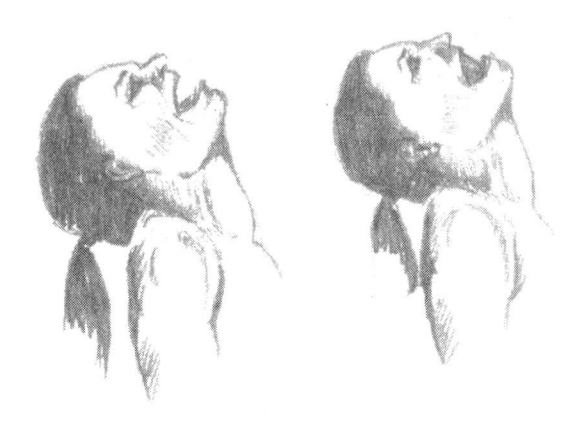

- **What is The Chin Up?** The Chin Up strengthening exercise targets the frontal muscles. It uses the muscle insertion points at the chin and the collarbone to provide an intense, area specific workout. Think of abdominal crunches – the Chin Up is the neck crunches of the neck strengthening world.

- **How do you do The Chin Up?** In your Neutral Zone, lift your chin up to the sky and lift your lower jaw up and down, for a count of ten. Bring your head back down and breathe, this is half of one set. For the next half, you are going to lift your chin back up to the sky, but this time touch the tip of your tongue to the roof of your mouth. Again lift your lower jaw up and down, for a count of ten and breathe. This was one set of the Chin Up, do three complete sets. Bringing the tip of your tongue up to the roof of your mouth strengthens the deeper muscles in your neck.

- **Why is The Chin Up Important?** This strengthening exercise targets the exact neck muscles that tend to sag and wrinkle under the chin. It works these muscles so they become firm and lean. Bringing you tongue up to the roof of your mouth adds an even deeper, more internal challenge to muscles and ligaments that are rarely strengthened in this way.

The Forward/Back Push

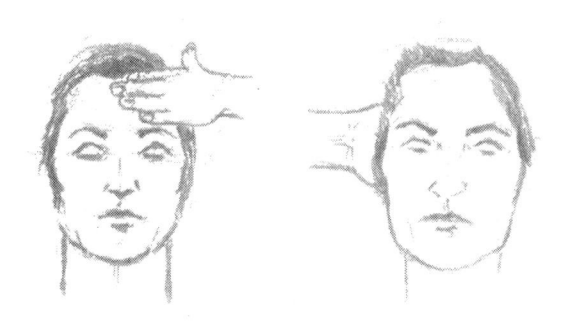

- **What is The Forward/Back Push?** This isometric exercise uses the resistance of three fingers to create tension within the neck muscles. No movement is required as in an isotonic exercise. The resistance created by the three fingers is enough to tone and strengthen the neck muscles.

- **How do you do The Forward/Back Push?** With your head straight, chin parallel to the floor, place three fingers on your forehead. You will be adding gentle resistance to this strengthening exercise. Now gently push your head against your three fingers and count to ten, forgetting not to breathe. Now place your three fingers on the back of your head and push your head against your fingers. Count to ten. This is one set, do three sets.

- **Why is The Forward/Back Push Important?** This particular isometric strengthening exercise utilizes muscles on many levels. Deep, internal muscles are activated as the resistance is applied. This deep tension is required to firm and strengthen all neck muscles. The next strengthening exercise – the Side to Side Push – will balance the Forward/Back Push.

The Side to Side Push

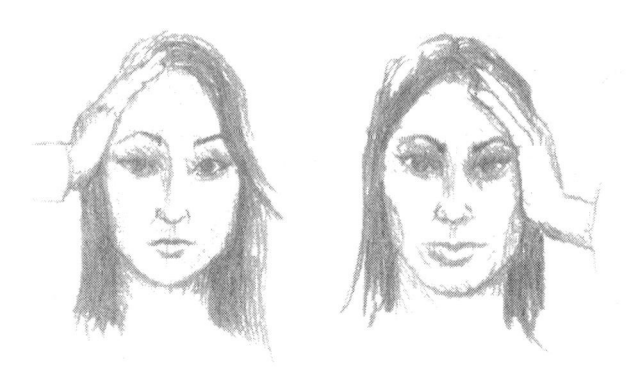

- **What is The Side to Side Push?** This isometric exercise balances the previous Forward/Back Push strengthening exercise. It targets the deep, internal side neck muscles that were not challenged by the resistance of the Forward/Back Push.

- **How do you do The Side to Side Push?** With the same head position in the Neutral Zone and the same three finger resistance, we will be going side to side. Place your three fingers on the right side of your head, above your temples. Now push to the right, counting to ten. Rest and repeat on the left side of your head, forgetting not to breathe. This is one set, do three sets.

- **Why is The Side to Side Push Important?** The neck is a complex, complete unit that works as one. We need to target and challenge all muscle groups if we are going to fight the effects of aging, namely the turkey or tech neck.

The Chin Tuck

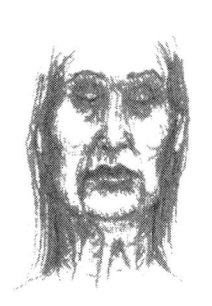

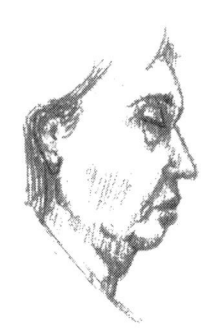

- **What is The Chin Tuck?** The Chin Tuck is a wonderfully powerful, subtle strengthening exercise! This is my personal favorite and I practice it ALL the time - when I'm eating, talking, standing, working, even before I fall asleep, I make a conscious effort to tuck my chin into my neck. The subtly of the Chin Tuck lies in the automatic movement the head has to take when the chin is tucked in – it is forced into the Neutral Zone. No more Forward Head Posture!

- **How do you do The Chin Tuck?** With your shoulders down and back, tuck your chin into your neck and count to five, breathe and return to the neutral position. Repeat three times.

- **Why is The Chin Tuck Important?** This is a very important exercise because it is your number one weapon against the Forward Head Posture. It is so simple and so easy to do that you can do it anywhere, any time. Tucking your chin in, automatically relaxes the cervical vertebrae, the back of the neck, causing them to align back into their natural, Neutral Zone. It also causes the head to lift up slightly, giving you a boost of confidence! Try to incorporate the Chin Tuck into every aspect of your daily life. You will instantly feel the benefits.

- **Total Strengthening Time:** 2 minutes.

Chapter Six: Children and Mobile Devices

It's not what you achieve, it's who you become - H.D. Thoreau

Turkey neck or even tech neck is not of great concern to a five or twelve year old child. But the parents of that five, twelve or sixteen year old should be concerned with a possible humped back due to their mobile device usage. Children are growing and developing by leaps and bounds at this age. It is important that growing children develop a good, strong posture. It is this good posture and healthy mobile device habits that will carry them through their lives.

With the introduction of technology and the mobile device world, the very concepts of flexibility and strength are becoming more and more of a challenge in a child's life. As adults maneuver through the new world of hand held mobile devices, not only are we developing new, healthy mobile device habits, we need to practice these lessons daily and then be able to teach them to our children.

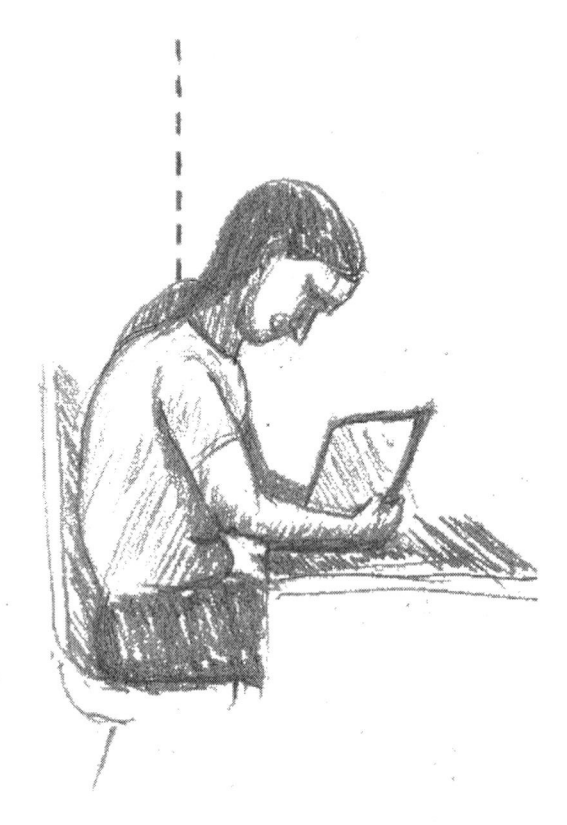

The average child wakes up usually with a hand held mobile device already in their hands. They go to school for eight hours and hopefully participate in a period of PE – physical education where they are physically challenging their bodies. They've probably spent their lunch period on their mobile devices, but hopefully they socialized, face-to-face with their friends. After school, they hopefully participate in an after school program, but probably go home and socialize/play games on their mobile devices. At dinner, hopefully there is interaction with the family unit. After dinner is homework, socializing, playing games, or watching a movie on their tablet or their phone.

The point of this scenario is not the fact that hand held mobile devices have infiltrated all stratospheres of our child's lives. This fact is here to stay! **But the sheer amount of time and the potential for poor posture is my concern.** Unfortunately the hand held mobile device industry has grown so rapidly, there are really no accessories or supportive devices out there yet. So until supportive devices are invented, self-awareness and self-correction have to be taught to our children and practiced by the whole family.

An article from The Daily Mail Online published in February 2014 followed a typical teenager Ryan, age 15 who was recently diagnosed with a "computer hump".

He spends up to 4 hours a day playing games and is being treated by Dr. Robin Lansman an Osteopath in England. Dr. Lansman said that in recent years he now sees at least one teenager a week with the same deformity.

The article goes on to discuss that researchers predict a "healthcare time bomb" of back and neck troubles among British youngsters, linked to the use of computers, video games and smartphones. Almost three-quarters of primary school children and nearly two-thirds of secondary school pupils interviewed told researches that they had suffered back or neck pain during the previous year, although 90% of them said that they had not told anyone about their discomfort.

Dr. Lansman noted that "in the worst case scenario, left untreated, it requires surgery. A metal rod is inserted in the spine which acts like scaffolding, keeping the back straight." He goes on to say that "computer hump develops when the spine becomes stiff and the ribcage is compressed from sitting stooped forward for long periods of time. We've been seeing it in adults for years but it's becoming increasingly common in teenagers. And the danger of it happening at such a young age, when you haven't reached your full height, is that the spine will grow out of shape, making it harder to straighten". Dr. Lansman treated Ryan over three months last year, manipulating the curvature in his spine and the muscles around it, to help smooth out his back. Ryan said "thankfully my back is less painful and not as warped since I started sitting properly and doing the exercises."

Exercise Five

Children, no matter their age, are aware of their bodies and what feels right. Older children are acutely aware of their appearance and body. Are your children living in the Neutral Zone? When they play on their tablets or on their video games, do they play in good posture? Do they know what good posture is and why it is important? This exercise will look outside of yourself and to your children, or any kids that are in your life – students, nieces, nephews or cousins – are they living in the Neutral Zone? Is your house Neutral Zone friendly? Do you have sofas and chairs that support the back? Do you have lots of pillows and throw blankets that can be used to support your mobile devices?

Our children have the world at their fingertips. They have the answer to any question, at any moment they desire. If you believe that knowledge is power, then this generation is a very powerful one indeed. So what role does a parent or teacher play in this new age of mobile device technology and their child? I believe that we really have nothing to teach them, as far as technology is concerned. In fact, they are pretty good at teaching us what is going on. What we can offer them is an explanation of why certain information is important to them, for example healthy mobile device habits. How this information can be implemented into their daily lives. And why this information, i.e. healthy mobile device habits is important to their lives. Children are bombarded by information and knowledge every day, all day. All that we can really do is offer them our wisdom as to why this information is important to their lives and how they can implement this knowledge safely.

As far as their posture and preventing humped backs is concerned, parents have the opportunity to act as a role model. When children see their parents operating in the Neutral Zone, taking time out to stretch and strengthen their necks, children will also follow. Teachers have the opportunity to incorporate these three steps into their physical or health education, or into a computer class. If children hear and see these healthy mobile device habits at home and then hear the same message at school, this would be a powerful teaching tool! Parents and teachers also need to be on the lookout for signs and symptoms of a more serious problem, caused by poor posture and long hours on hand held mobile devices.

Dr. Hansraj, the New York City chief of spine surgery stated in his latest article *Assessment of Stresses in the Cervical Spine Caused by Posture and Position of the Head* that "people spend an average of two to four hours a day with their heads tilted over reading and texting on their smart phones and devices.

Cumulatively this is 700 to 1400 hours a year of excess stresses seen about the cervical spine. It is possible that a high school student may spend an extra 5,000 hours in poor posture." It is "the extra 5,000" hours that is alarming and needs to brought into the consciousness of society. The best tool to address this potential crisis is acceptance and adoption of healthy mobile device habits. Not only do parents and teachers need to be good role models, they also need to be aware of signs and symptoms of poor posture children assume while using their hand held mobile devices.

Some warning signs of serious postural issues may include, but not limited to:

- Headaches, is your child holding his or her head, sensitive to light or loud noise?
- Sore eyes, is she or he squinting and rubbing her eyes?
- Neck and/or back pain
- Tingling in the arms of fingers

These are signs that need to be addressed by your health care provider.

The goal of this book is to be used as a preventive tool, a simple tool to prevent the above problems from even occurring. With the use of the Neutral Zone, the stretches and strengthening exercises, these problems will hopefully be avoided. But if these signs and symptoms are present in your child, there may already be underlying problems that must be addressed by a healthcare provider.

How can we teach children healthy mobile device habits?

- Teach and reflect the importance of the Neutral Zone and good posture during mobile device usage. Explain why this is important to them. Older children are concerned about their appearance and will be open to these teachings.
- Teach and reflect techniques of maintaining good posture, for example using pillows or toys for the younger children to hold up and support their mobile devices. Always support the back if sitting and if standing,

bend the elbows and lift the mobile device up to eye level.

- Be aware of the time spent on their mobile device and after twenty minutes, teach children to take a break, or to take a few minutes to stretch their neck and check their posture.
- Talk and teach openly about the side effects of poor posture and using their mobile devices and the importance of telling an adult if they experience pain or discomfort.

Conclusion

We're still in the first minute of the first day of the Internet revolution - Scott Cook

The world of hand held mobile devices is a young world and still growing. Along with growth inevitably comes a few growing pains and I believe this book addresses an important and potentially dangerous growing pain – poor mobile device posture. Yes we can "just put our tablet down" and try to live a more balanced life, not so dependent on our devices, but personally I do not think this is realistic. Our mobile devices have become so important in our work, play, relaxation and socializing that even if we do attempt to live a "balanced life" it is going to include our mobile devices! What really needs to change is us on our mobile devices, beginning first and foremost with healthy mobile device habits.

The sole purpose of this book was to be used as a preventive tool, by becoming aware of and then developing healthy mobile device habits. The first preventive tool is the tool of self- awareness.

Awareness of ourselves and of our body posture as we are using our hand held mobile devices, and the awareness of keeping our bodies in the low stress, no distress zone known as the Neutral Zone. The second tool is stretching our necks at least once a day and after twenty minutes of solid mobile devices usage. The last important tool would be strengthening the neck muscles at least once a day, keeping our neck muscles firm, developed and strong.

Preventive tools are only helpful if practiced and used on a regular daily basis. Like a seat belt, it can only work when you use it every time you sit in a car. In order to fight the aging effects of mobile devices, we need to correct our poor posture and neglected muscles and tendons that cause turkey neck and a humped back. Another very important preventive point was shared in Gray's Anatomy under the *Chemical Composition of Muscle* section. It states that "in chemical composition, the muscular fibres may be said, in round numbers, to consist of 75 percent of water, about 20 percent of proteids, 2 percent of fat, 1 percent of nitrogenous extractives and carbohydrates and 2 percent of salts which is mainly potassium phosphate and carbonate." Our muscles need water and lots of it to stay young. Other preventive tools for healthy neck muscles are:

- Getting eight hours of sound sleep and using a supportive pillow for our necks
- Healthy diet and maintaining a healthy weight
- Sunscreen the face and neck by day and moisturize the face and neck by night
- Practice the Alexander Technique all day, everyday
- Practice the Neutral Zone at all times, but especially when using your mobile devices
- Do the toilet test daily and stretch and strengthen there too – it works!!

In a perfect world, we work for eight hours a day, we play for eight hours a day and we sleep for eight hours a day. Hand held mobile devices have become an important part of our work and play time, and with the introduction of fitness bands, we are now relying on this mobile device to let us know how we slept, how many hours of deep sleep we had and what our blood pressure and heart rate was, during our sleep time. We need our mobile devices 24/7! I believe this is a wonderful thing. The more information we have at our disposal, the better choices we can make. And the more that we can learn about ourselves, the easier we can see our unhealthy choices and fix or make better ones. As we learned from Dr. Hansraj's study *Assessment of Stresses in the Cervical Spine Caused by Posture and Position of the Head,* "people spend an average of two to four hours a day with their heads tilted over reading and texting on their smart phones and devices. Cumulatively this is 700 to 1400 hours a year of excess stresses seen about the cervical spine. It is possible that a high school student may spend an extra 5,000 hours in poor posture." (Surgical Technology International XXV) Those "extra 5,000 hours in poor posture" is the reason that this preventive book is needed at this time. If you consider all of the new video gaming and new apps coming out, targeting our children, an extra 5,000 hours a year becomes even more realistic. Let's take a quick look at exactly how long "an extra 5,000 hours" on top of the typical 1,400 hours of mobile device usage looks like. Suppose you are one of the lucky ones that get to sleep eight hours a night. In one year, you will have slept 2,688 hours. That is just over half of the time kids spend on their devices. Or suppose a child goes to school for eight hours and then does their homework and helps mom and dad around the house for another eight hours – every day of the week – that would total 5,376 hours a year! This is where the "potential national healthcare crisis" that the chiropractor Dr. Lansman in England mentioned and is so concerned about.

So not only is living and practicing healthy mobile device habits important, reflecting and mirroring them to our children is even more important. This is the generation that will be taking the mobile device world into its next generation. So let's teach them how to do this in a healthy and smart way. Other points that were touched upon for children and worth repeating here:

- Practice and reflect healthy mobile device habits around the house
- Teach children why the Neutral Zone, stretching and strengthening are important, especially for their still developing bodies

- Teach children the signs and symptoms of possible health problems due to poor posture while on their mobile devices
- Teach children why these signs and symptoms are important to know and why they need to tell their parents or their school nurse.

Acknowledgments

The author would like to thank the following people: Tracy for all the smiles and never ending support, Frank at SBCS for helping me see the business of writing, Angela and Todd at BookLocker.com, Inc., Dr. Ralph at AIDO Health Center for his professional advice and guidance, Barbara McNichols and her editing skills, Delores and allowing me to check in – thank you, Gwendolen for her inspiration and girl power and mostly for the Universal Guidance and Love and shining of Light onto words – thank you.